MAXWELL POWER

Fitness For People with No TIme

How to squeeze exercise into your already busy life.

To my son .

*Every minute of life is priceless
and will never be repeated, so
take time to enjoy, be grateful
for, and celebrate your existence.
I love you.*

The key to building good habits is to start
small and make them easy to do.

James Clear

Contents

Acknowledgement

I want to thank Holy Athletes for their daily inspiration.

Instagram

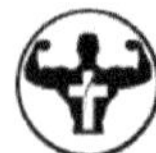

holy.athletes

Follow   **Message**

Holy Athletes
Community
✝ | Daily Motivation and Scriptures
✝ | With God all things are possible!!
✝ | Follow us on TikTok & Twitter in the highlights
below

TikTok   Twitter

1

Introduction

My lifelong wiry build of 5' 10" and 160 lbs, nearly impossible to put on body mass, was chalked up to an incredibly high metabolism. I was active, played sports, worked out, and generally felt good about myself. I still had a flat stomach and defined, albeit small, muscles.

Years later, staring in the mirror, I couldn't believe what or even who I was looking at. Was this me? It didn't look like me at all. I had a belly so big I could barely see the tips of my toes. The start of a double chin had emerged, and I felt weak, slow, and highly out of shape. All I could think about while looking at this stranger in the mirror was, how did this happen? How did I go from an energetic, wiry twenty-something to this overweight 185 lb. blob seemingly overnight?

As my career progressed and I started a family, I had less time for activities like golf and softball, and found it harder to find time to work out. The trifecta of bad eating habits, lack of Fitness, and my mental habits changed utterly. The less "perceived time I had," the more weight I gained and the worse I felt, leading to less activity because it was more challenging. Pizza and pasta were a staple for me at least four to five days a week. I stopped going to the gym completely. Aside from the little walking I did throughout my typical day at work, I stopped all physical activity.

If any of this sounds familiar, the feeling of not having time to do the things you love to do, much less exercise, this book will address the barriers preventing you from achieving your full potential head-on. It will also give you strategies to overcome the excuses holding you hostage to inactivity and help you build lasting habits so Fitness becomes a part of your routine (again.) Lastly, I will review three powerful yet time-saving workouts to help you get into better shape with all the time constraints you may have in your busy life. So let's get started on this journey to a better you.

2

Objections

Welcome to Fitness for People with No Time. My name is Maxwell Power, and you're reading this book because you, like me, have struggled to add a fitness regime to your busy life. How often do people make New Year's resolutions that have lasted only a few weeks or months? Typically, January and February are the busiest months for new gym memberships. If you've belonged to one, you know they become less crowded as the Year drags on. It's easy for people to fall back into their pre-New Year's resolution routines and not build new and lasting habits. Why? Because people generally don't like change, and secondly, you have to spend hours in the gym every week to achieve anything; at least that's what the fitness magazines tell us. Not to mention the daily distractions creep in, and there are many reasons our new habits fall off or are only partially ingrained.

Why don't we work out consistently? Excuses, excuses, excuses. "I hate exercising," "I don't have the time," "I'm too tired," "It's too painful," "I have an injury," "I'm too old," "I'm embarrassed to exercise," and "I'm already in pretty good shape" to name some. Why do we make excuses, and more importantly, why do we let them prohibit us from reaching

3

our goals? The world-renowned guru to the stars, Tony Robbins, preaches, "Most people would rather avoid pain, working out, than gain pleasure, seeing the results of working out. It's easy to make excuses, but the fact of the matter is it's not easy to ingrain new habits. American entrepreneur Orrin Woodward says, "You must be willing to do what others **won't** if you want to accomplish what others **don't**." That's true in business, in sports, and, of course, in Fitness. This book will look at what small steps we can take daily to overcome these excuses, but let's look at some of the distractions holding us back.

- *Make a list of your top 3 - 5 excuses you make for yourself not to exercise consistently.*

One of the biggest culprits is T.V. With Netflix, Paramount + & Disney +, to name a few; these studios all create some of the most captivating programming since the advent of television. Couple that with the fact that everyone around us is talking about the latest series, shows or movies, and it's hard <u>not</u> to get sucked into watching to see for yourself or be part of the conversation. It doesn't take much effort to relax on the couch and passively get lost in the theater of our homes. I'm not saying we should stop watching T.V. altogether, but we are all guilty of watching way more than we think we do.

Another culprit is Social Media. One of the biggest challenges in raising kids (mine are now in their teens and early twenties) is to limit their exposure to electronics and social media. Did you ever sit down and say, I'm just going to watch a few videos on Instagram or YouTube, only to realize later that you've been on your phone for an hour and maybe two? Rarely are we on social media to accomplish something productive. More often than not, it's to see what friends and family, celebrities, etc., are doing. The psychological effects of prolonged exposure to social media have been well documented. Still, aside from that, it wastes precious time when we could be doing something good for our well-being.

- *Keep track of how many minutes you watch T.V., surf the internet, and spend on your phone looking at social media sites each day for a week. You'll probably be shocked at the number you record.*

Certain people in your life may also contribute to the distraction of not creating new and good habits. In this case, it is not that they are against you taking on your new fitness regime, but that fitness regime gets in the way of spending time with them in your life. I will discuss this in a later chapter regarding who should know about your exercise goals vs. who you should tell about your "give up" goals (like smoking.)

Everyone is busy, tired, distracted, afraid of failure, and we don't like to be uncomfortable or feel discomfort (pain from working out.) Inevitably, we listen to all those objections and take them as the truth. We are our own worst enemy when it comes to building new habits. Looking objectively at the two lists you will be making (mentioned above), we should start to understand how much time we spend on things that may not be in our best interest. I'm not saying you can't watch TV or surf the internet to get into a good fitness habit; I am telling you to understand how much you spend on these distractions. The next chapter will delve into how to overcome these self-inflicted objections.

3

Objections No More

S o, let's look at some objections and how to handle them. I get overwhelmed thinking about the time it will take to work out. Rome wasn't built in a day, and neither will your new body. One way to overcome this is by starting small. In his #1 New York Times Best Selling Book "Atomic Habits' James Clear talks about improving by 1% daily. If you improve by a small fraction each day, you may not notice anything the first week, month, or even six months, but over the long run, you will be amazed at how much stronger you will become. If, however, you decline by 1% a day and do things that are counterproductive to your fitness goals, it creeps up on you without you even noticing.

The one positive I can take away from the pandemic in 2019 was creating a new daily yoga habit for myself. I downloaded the Peloton App on my phone to do yoga daily. So excited, I went to the app and started with a 30-minute beginner class. I barely got through it; I was sweating profusely, my body was screaming for me to stop (I was very inflexible at that point,) and I could barely do the beginner poses for half the time allotted in the training. I was so down on myself that I almost canceled the yearly subscription after that first day.

I regrouped the following day and said my new mantra: "This is not a sprint; it's a marathon." I'm not going to be as flexible as Gumby overnight. So, on day 2, I started with just a 10-minute beginner class. I repeated the same class for two weeks until I felt more confident with my balance and holding the poses. I increased to a 15-minute class the following week and eventually worked my way up to 30 minutes, and on days/weekends when the time was allotted, I did an hour of beginner class. I sprinkled in restorative yoga (more of a meditation than poses) on the days my body didn't feel up to it. Within six months, I became more flexible. I built a new habit that, instead of dreading, as I did when I started, became my escape and an activity I genuinely look forward to. Lesson learned is that I started small. Even 5 minutes a day to keep moving will help you build your new fitness regime.

- Key takeaway: Listen to what your body is telling you as you start your new venture.

When your barrier is, "Why am I putting myself through this [torture]? You have to change your mindset and words to describe the activity. You don't HAVE to work out; you GET to work out. I remember having a conversation with my Dad a few weeks before he passed. At this point, he was home in hospice, and I asked him, if he were granted one wish, what would it be? He thought momentarily and said, "I would love just to walk again. I would love to walk along the beach with your mother. I'd spend the entire day just walking and talking." The sad reality is that no matter what age you are, we will not be able to do what we can today. Change your feeling toward this new activity and take advantage of what your body can give you TODAY! Working out is a way to love yourself, better your health, and better your life. 1 Corinthians 3:16-17 says, "Don't you know that you are God's temple and that God's Spirit dwells in your midst?" You only get one body; it's never too late to start caring for it. Remember that every morning, you wake up.

A 2016 *Wall Street Journal* article states, "The most successful, and therefore productive, people typically rise at 4 am." It may make sense because only a few people in your circle of friends and family are up at that time, reducing distractions you may have later in the day. One caveat to this is that we all need our sleep. According to *Matthew Solan, Executive Editor of Harvard Men's Health Watch*, the average American needs 7 hours of sleep. Some need a little more, and some require a little less, so if you plan on waking up early to start your new fitness habit, plan accordingly and start going a little earlier than you're used to. Suppose you continue to stay up as usual and wake up an hour or two earlier. In that case, that is a recipe for stalling in your new habit before it starts. Takeaway: get the sleep your body needs as you take on your new exercise regimen.

Who should you tell about your new desire to get fit? The late, great motivational speaker Zig Ziglar, whom I had the pleasure of having dinner within the mid '90s, said if it's a "give up a goal" or something you're quitting, feel free to tell the world about it. The more people know what you're trying to give up, the better because they will help keep you on track. But if it's a "Go up goal," something you're trying to accomplish, like, in this case, building a new habit of Fitness in your life, be very selective about who you tell. You only want to share with those who will be 100% supportive of your goal. If you tell everyone about your "go up" goal may lead to more barriers to sticking with your plan.

So, the most challenging part of building any new habit or routine is getting started. The more you can consistently stick with it, usually seeing results, the easier it is to maintain. In his 1960 Bestselling book Psycho-Cybernetics, plastic surgeon Maxwell Maltz claimed it took 21 days to get used to the new you after plastic surgery, get used to a new house, and even change new beliefs. So don't expect to fully embrace your new Fitness routine right away. Furthermore, a 2009 study on forming new habits concluded that it takes anywhere from 18 days to 254 days to create a new habit, with a reported average of about 66 days. What does all this mean for those of us starting a new exercise routine? Everyone is different, and habit forming comes in many different time frames. Still, the bottom line is that the pain of quitting before the habit is formed is far outweighed by the health benefits of pushing through to form a new habit in the first place. No matter what the obstacle or what excuse your mind dreams up, the only way to break through and form your new habit is to **not give up**. If you find yourself on a day you just can't get motivated, ***don't beat yourself up***. Start the next day, even if it's a modified workout, but you must get back on the horse.

To overcome the barriers preventing you from becoming the best you can be, you need to recognize the distractions and change how you feel about them to overcome them. In his article Overcoming Our Biggest Obstacle to Creating Habits, Leo Babauta says you have to have answers to the objections you make up in your head. When you say to yourself, "I'm too tired, do __________," no matter how little effort you give, give it effort. It could be the first one or two of the exercises of the programs outlined below, or it's to go outside for a 10-minute brisk walk, but whatever the task, do it. Afterward, you will truly feel like you've accomplished something.

4

Time Management Strategies

I f long "to-do" lists are overwhelming and cumbersome, try filling out the "Time management matrix" below. This four-quadrant strategy enables you to take a good hard look at your daily/weekly/monthly activities so you can visualize and understand what's important, not necessary, urgent, and not urgent in your life right now. This will help you focus on what you need to spend most of your free time accomplishing. I learned a lot about where I was spending my time after I filled this out. I encourage you to print out the PDF version and fill it out before you move on to the next chapter.

The Time Management Matrix

	Urgent	Not Urgent
Important	1 2 3 4 5 6 7 8 9 10	1 2 3 4 5 6 7 8 9 10
Not Important	1 2 3 4 5 6 7 8 9 10	1 2 3 4 5 6 7 8 9 10

(Draw a similar chart on a blank piece of paper and fill it out)

Here are some helpful tips on creating less chaos in your life. Do this now!

- Turn off all the notifications on your phone. This will reduce distractions throughout your day as well as the temptation to be on it and get sucked into the social media vortex of procrastination.
- Set limits on television time and browsing your social media sites. Set aside a Time each day to do these things, and when you sit to do them, set a timer on your phone for your allowable daily amount. Be strict with this task; get up and be productive when the timer

goes off. This will free up dozens and dozens of hours over a few weeks and months.

5

The Importance of Goals

Setting goals for the things you want to achieve is easy, but not always as easy to stick with it or follow through to the end. A goal until you take action is just a "good idea." The entrepreneur in me has had so many ideas over the years, most of which I did nothing with. Some of them others thought of as well, and I know that, because they followed through on the idea.

My grandfather, trained early to be a butcher by his immigrant uncles in Rhode Island, He created a steak sauce when he was in his late teens and I can remember when I was young, he would make this sauce in huge pots on his stove in Brooklyn for friends and family. I would always ask him, "Pop, when will you bottle and sell this stuff? Everyone loves it." He would give me the same answer: anyone could make it.

Years later, in my twenties, I set a goal and started bottling this secret family recipe and selling it in New York. Initially, it was a lot of work, finding the right size bottle, making the labels, working with Cornell University's food science department to have all the correct nutritional information on the label, etc. I made it a point to put a little time and effort into it each day, around fifteen to twenty minutes. Then there was the selling part. Initially, it was a little nerve-wracking, but eventually, I became more comfortable and confident the more I sold. I had butcher shops, grocery stores, and hundreds of private customers that I would sell directly to. None of this would have ever happened if I didn't take action. The story's point is that you must take **daily** action on your goals, even small ones.

With goal setting, you want to be realistic with your goals. Some may be saying if Roger Bannister, the first man to run a sub-four minute mile competitively, was realistic about his goals, he may have yet to achieve the unthinkable. Agreed, but the key to goals is to attain small achievable goals in the beginning to build the confidence to continue with loftier goals.

The acronym stands for Specific, Measurable, Achievable, Relevant & Time-Based. The more specific, the more focused you will be on them and the likelihood you will attain them. It takes time for a new goal to be accepted by your brain before it becomes a habit. For everyone, that time frame may be different. Be patient and stick with it. Positive affirmations said daily out loud is a great way to continue to train your brain to build new habits. Repeat your goal to yourself in the mirror or driving your car. Your goal must come from you, not from someone else.

Examples of affirmations you can use:

- "I stick to my goals and achieve them."
- "I love how I feel after a great workout."
- "I look, feel, and sound great this morning."
- "When people see me smile, they can't help but smile too."

Add your own to this list, write them out, and post them on your bathroom mirror.

6

Celebrating Milestones

So you've decided to add Fitness into your busy life and set some goals; now what? One of the simple ways to stay focused and continue or build on your recent successes is to recognize your accomplishments. This is important because it keeps you motivated to achieve the next goal or compound the one you have just achieved. Tony Robbins gives practical ways to celebrate your small (or significant) achievements.

- Spend time with loved ones.
- Show your appreciation to those supporting you through the process.
- Practice gratitude. Start a gratitude journal and write every day, even if it's only for 3 minutes.
- Be spontaneous. Go out to dinner, hike, and make plans with friends.
- Use it to fuel you. Look at yourself in the mirror and tell yourself how great you are. You have only scratched the surface. Where will you be a year from now?

Do not skip this important step of your journey. It's gonna take a lot of commitment and small actions every day to achieve your new goal of incorporating Fitness into your busy life, celebrate the small successes you have along the way.

When I coached my kids growing up in all the sports they played, some of the best moments was at the end of practice or a game, where we celebrated a player for their achievements in that practice. The simple acknowledgment went a long way for the players confidence and drive to continue to improve. Whether is adding fitness into your life for 3 straight day, even for ten minutes, acknowledge to yourself the small achievement you just hit. Again, you will not see miraculous changes in your physique on a daily or monthly basis, but you will be improving the 1% to instill new habits and create a lasting change to your health and well being.

7

Why Walking?

S o, you've committed to changing your life and adding Fitness and a healthier lifestyle to your daily routine. How can we do this painlessly and effectively? It's not just the three workouts outlined in the next chapters, but there is an easy, low-impact activity we can do daily to increase our well-being, self-esteem, and confidence. Let's look at some strategies you can start incorporating today or tomorrow. :-)

Walking daily is a great way to raise your heart rate and improve your cardiovascular system. You may be wondering how long I have to walk for it to be considered exercise Isn't. This is counterproductive to why I am reading your book on Fitness for people who need more time. It only takes 10-15 minutes of brisk walking to raise your heart rate and has equivalent effects to running. In a 2013 meta-analysis study that included close to 50,000 patients, the results were as stated: Equivalent energy expenditures by moderate walking and vigorous running exercise produced similar risk reductions for hypertension, high cholesterol, diabetes, and possibly coronary heart disease.

How do I increase the amount I walk daily without adding more time for Fitness to my schedule? One way is always to opt to take the stairs vs the elevator. This is a great way to increase the number of daily steps and the added benefit of the energy expended in your legs to climb the flight(s) you encounter. With the advent of smartwatches, counting the number of daily steps is easy. A great goal is 10,000 steps per day, which astonishingly is about a 5-mile walk. You'd be surprised how much you do or don't walk when you keep track. Don't have a smartphone, you can pick up a cheap pedometer (step counter) online for $2-$5. Carol Welch, Doctor of Physical Therapy, said is best, "Movement is a medicine for creating change in a person's physical, emotional and mental states."

I recently watched the documentary *Live to 100 secrets of the Blue Zones*. When they went on location in Sardinia Italy there was a strong correlation between how steep the streets the centenarians walked up each day top get to town to how long they lived. The steeper the hill, the more cardiovascular exercise they achieved and the longer they lived. Unfortunately we all don't live in a town built on mountains like they have in Europe, so we have to do our best to walk as much as we can. Think of the centenarians when you decide to take the elevator or escalator the next time your out an about. Take the advice from the little blue fish Dori from Finding Nemo when she said, "Just keep swimming [moving], swimming [moving], swimming [moving.]"

8

1 The Body Weight Workout

For those who have not been part of an exercise program for a long time, it could be an overwhelming and daunting task to even think about. In this chapter, I will go over exercises you can do right now, no matter how old you are. Welcome to body weight exercises. These exercises can be performed in the comfort of your home without buying expensive equipment or joining a gym. Although the following exercises seem pretty basic, depending on your shape, they may be challenging initially, but remember, that's a good thing.

The key to these exercises is not to overdo it, but instead make sure you're building on what you have accomplished the week before. The beauty of this workout is that the resistance comes from your body. As you become stronger, you will start to build "lean body muscle" and lose some excess fat you may be carrying around? This is a great exercise program for those with no time because you don't have the burden of getting in your car to go to a gym. This program will improve your balance, flexibility, and strength. For the first week, if you can only do 3-5 reps for each exercise, that's OK. Listen to your body and then build from there.

Body Weight Exercises:

Mountain climbers - Like the name, this is the movement we will mimic. This is a great exercise to warm your body for the exercises to follow. This exercise will work most of the muscles in your body, including your legs, core, triceps, and shoulders. Get in the push up position (at the top of the push up) and alternate, bringing your knees to your chest.

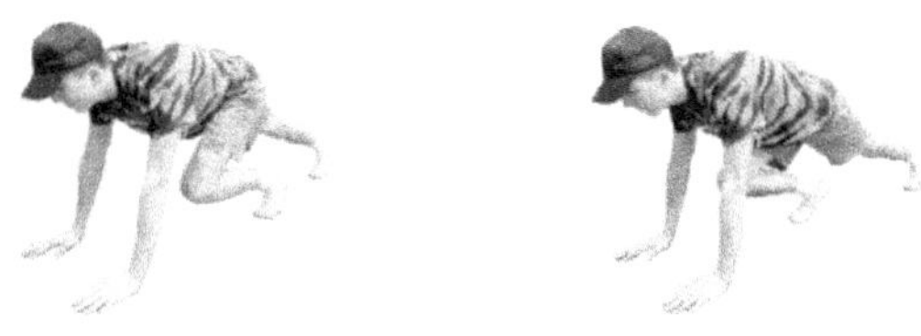

Push ups - This exercise works not only your chest and triceps to push your body up off the ground but also your shoulders and your abdominal, which work to keep your core tight. This is one of the best body weight exercises you can do for your upper body. You want to keep your back straight, using your abdominal muscles, and not let your chest, midsection, or legs touch the ground at the bottom of the rep. Another good rule of thumb is to do each push up, or rep, slowly and in control. Don't give in or give up. Even if you can only do 1, 2, or 3 push ups the first day you start, strive to do the same number of reps each day for a week and build on the number the next week.

Air Squats - This is a great exercise to build lower body strength and flexibility in both your legs and hips. This exercise works all the lower body muscles, including your quadriceps (big muscles on your upper leg), Hamstrings (muscles on the back of your legs), hip abductors (muscles by your hip and smaller muscles of your butt), and gluteus maximus (the most significant muscle of the buttocks)

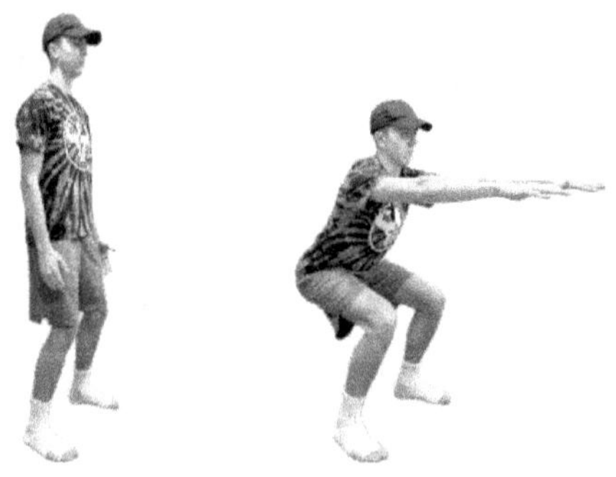

Planks - Great static (lack of movement) exercise to strengthen your core or abdominal area. The added benefit of strengthening these muscles is that it will help reduce back pain. Get into the position and hold for 30 seconds. Build on that weekly.

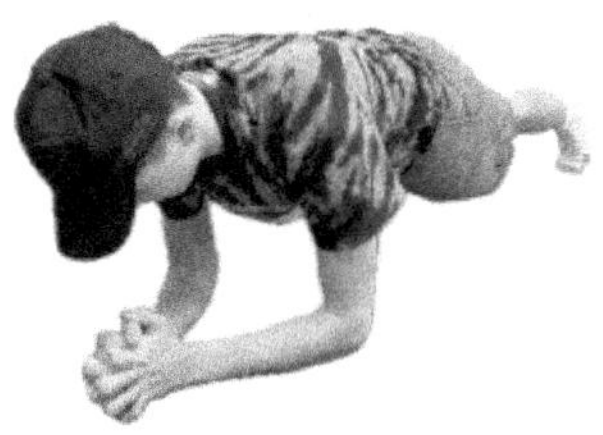

Lunges - Great exercise to continue to strengthen your legs and core. Start standing straight with feet shoulder-width apart—hands on hips, with elbows pointing to the sides. Start with one foot and step forward, bending at the knee, making sure the knee doesn't go farther than your toes. Step back up to the starting position and alternate legs. Start with 10 reps each leg and build from there.

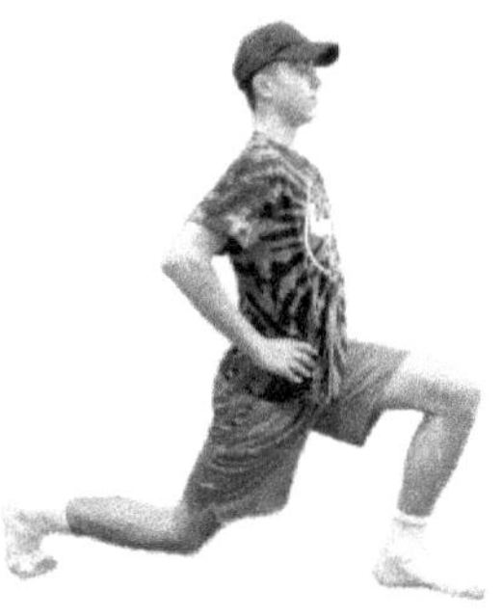

Abdominal crunch - Another important core exercise. Lie on your back with your knees bent and your heels close to your buttocks. Cross your arms in front of your chest with your hands resting opposite shoulders. Slowly and controlled, raise your upper back off the floor, feeling a tightening of your abdominal muscle (you only need to lift your shoulders an inch or two off the floor till you feel your core engaged). Hold for 5 seconds, and go back down slowly; once your shoulders lightly touch the ground, start the next repetition. Do this exercise for 30 seconds and build from there.

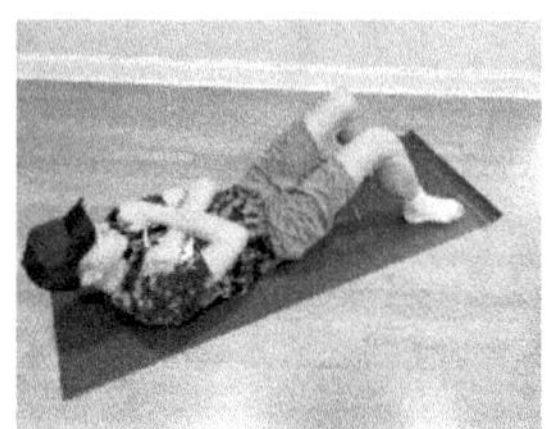

Stair step-ups - This is an excellent exercise for your glutes and hamstrings, as well as some cardio. Standing in front of a step, start with either foot, step onto the step, and load your weight onto the leg you stepped up on (what I mean by that is to put most of your weight on the front leg). If you do this correctly, you will not use the back leg (foot on the ground) to help push, so your front leg does 95% of the work. Keep your back leg (and foot) suspended in the air behind you throughout the step up and down. This is also a great exercise to work on balance. Start with just stepping up one step and increase to two after you have built the strength to do one step easily. (Don't recommend more than 2 steps, for balance reasons) Start with 10 step ups with each leg and build from there.

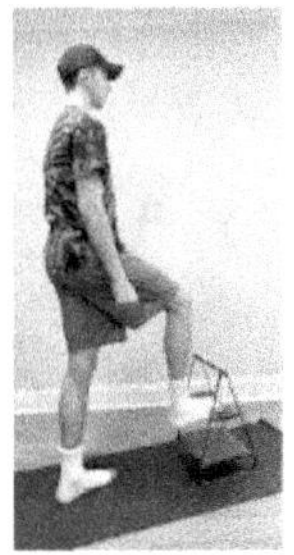 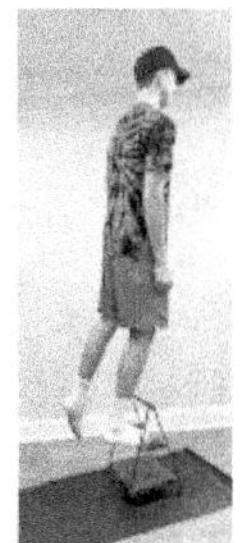

Superman - This is a great exercise to build strength in your lower back muscles and to help prevent back pain in the future. To do this, get into the bottom of a push up position and lie with your belly on a yoga mat, rug, or towel on the floor. To start the rep, lift your head off the ground, bring your elbows to the sky, which lifts your hands off the ground, pinching the middle of your upper back while raising your feet off the ground. Sounds complicated, but if done correctly, your lower abdomen and pelvis are the only areas contacting the ground. Note this was a challenging exercise when I started, so don't be discouraged if you can only do a few reps in the beginning, holding for only a second or two. Repeat this for ten reps. Over time, your lower back, upper legs, and core will strengthen to allow you to progress further with this exercise.

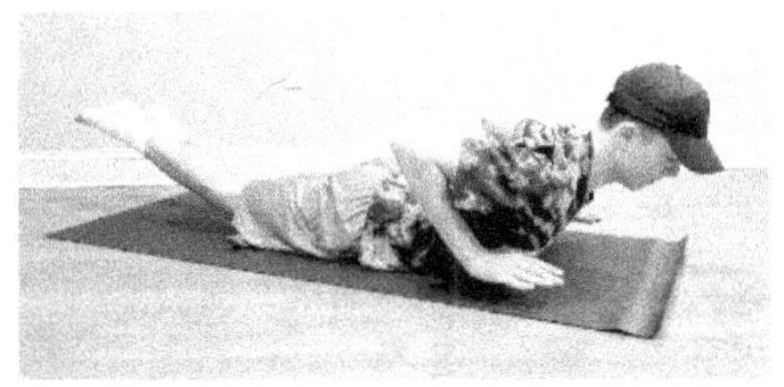

Pelvic Tilt - This is an excellent static exercise but very effective in strengthening your core—the same starting position at the abdominal crunch. Lie on your back with your knees bent and your heels close to your buttocks. Then, tighten your abdominal muscles, pulling your belly down to the floor and feeling your entire spine pressing against the floor. Hold for 5 seconds, release for 5 seconds, and repeat. Start with 5 to 10 reps and increase by a couple each week.

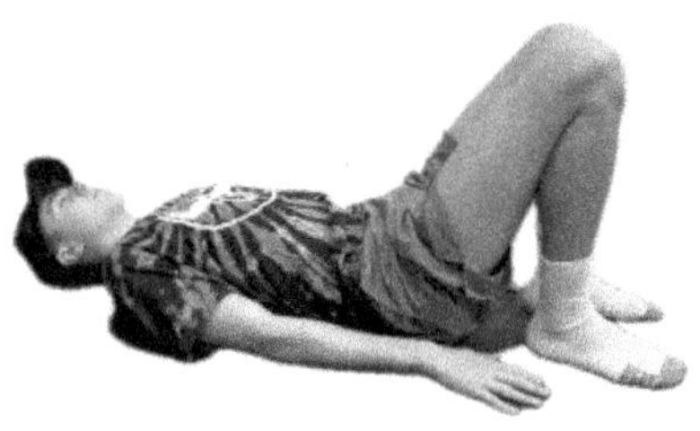

9

2 The Micro Workout

For years, we were told by trainers and fitness magazine articles that the way to build lean body muscle and put on mass was to spend hours in the gym and consume a high-calorie diet. Many workout programs look like this: spend 3 to 4 days in the gym for at least 60-90 minutes per workout, working a maximum of two muscle groups per session. Example: Day 1 Back & Biceps, Day 2 Chest and Triceps, Day 3 Shoulders & Legs. Finish all workouts with 30 minutes of cardio on the stationary bike, stair master, or treadmill. I'm overwhelmed writing these words, much less going to the gym to do it.

This is not the only way to build the critical lean body muscle needed to look good, feel good, and potentially extend our precious lives. Welcome to the Micro Workout. All you require is a set of dumbbells and you. Start dumbbells light enough to be able to safely lift over your head. Micro Workouts consist of 5-10 minute sessions, two to three times daily, activating your type II or "Fast twitch" muscles by performing short burst resistance training. The key is that you will be fresh with each session, maximizing your potential and working your muscles to the max.

When to do these micro workouts? Start in the morning after you get out of bed, if you can, before lunch, and then right before dinner each day. This schedule not only helps you manage your blood sugar and control your appetite, but it also allows your body to rest and recover before your next session so you can maximize muscle growth potential quickly. This routine has the bonus of maintaining a pump throughout the day, which may help build your confidence, self-esteem, and overall attitude.

Micro workout 1 of 3

Shoulder press / mini squat - 10-20 reps every minute for 5 minutes:m (morning)

1. Lift your dumbbells onto your shoulders, palms facing in. Take a breath and brace your core. First, dip at the knees and use your legs to help.
2. Then, press your dumbbells overhead. Lower under control to the ground. After ten reps, switch partners.

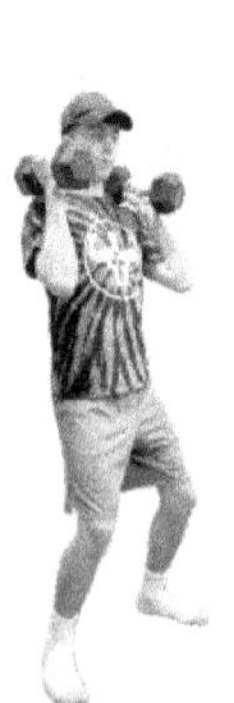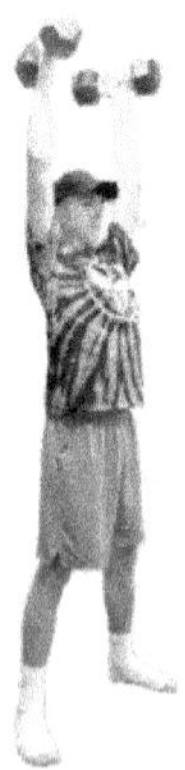

Push ups - 10-20 reps every minute for 5 minutes:

1. First, drop into a strong plank position, with your core tight and hands on your dumbbells.
2. Then bend your elbows to bring your chest to the floor. Keep your elbows close to your body as you push back up explosively.

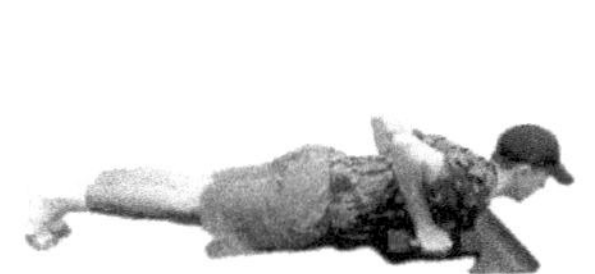 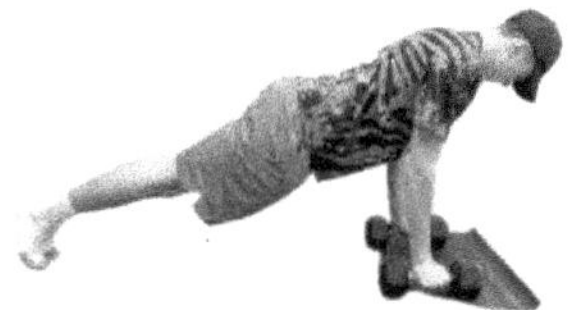

Micro workout 2 of 3

Front squats - 10-20 reps every minute for 5 minutes:(noon)

1. First, lift your dumbbells and secure them on your shoulders.
2. Then, from here, drop into a front squat until your thighs pass parallel to the ground, before driving back up. Fatigue will set in by this point, but focus on your breathing and keep your form tight.

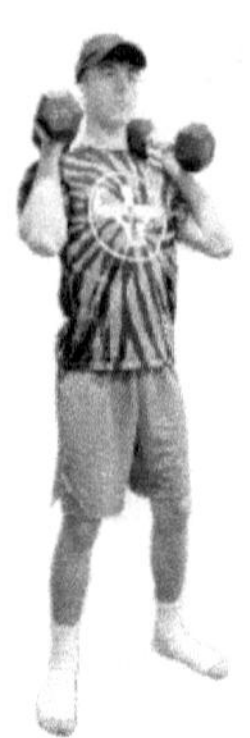 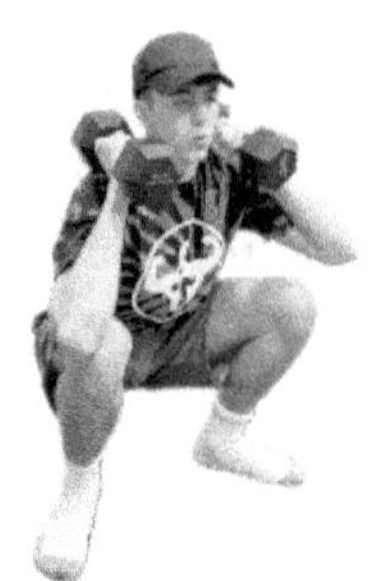

Dead lifts - 10-20 reps every minute for 5 minutes:

1. First, with your dumbbells on the floor just outside your feet, hinge down and grip them with a flat back and neutral spine.
2. Then, engage your lats and stand upright, pushing the ground away with your feet, keeping your chest and black flat throughout.
3. Lower them back to the ground in a hinging motion and repeat.

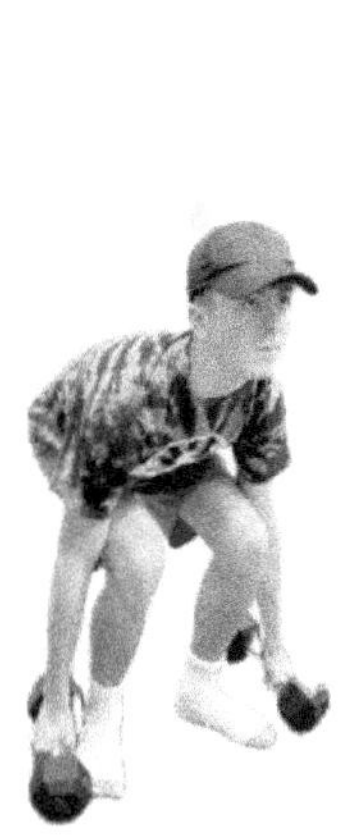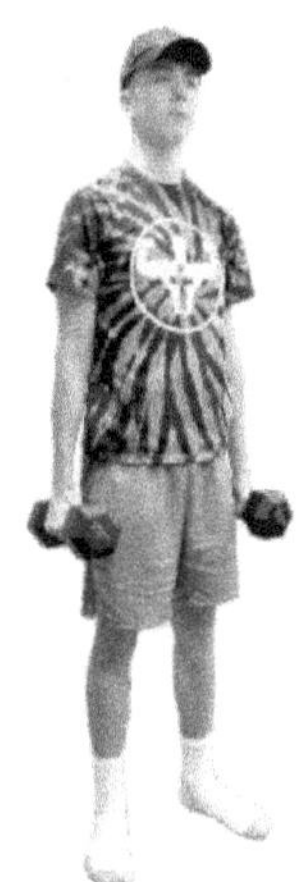

Micro Workout 3 of 3

Bent over rows - 10-20 reps every minute for 5 minutes: (night)

1. First hold your dumbbells at your sides and hinge at the hips until your chest is parallel to the floor, dumbbells hanging below your knees.
2. Then, keeping your elbows close to your body, row both dumbbells towards your hips, squeeze your shoulder blades down and together, and lower them under control to the start before repeating. Avoid using momentum from your torso and focus on squeezing your back rigidly.

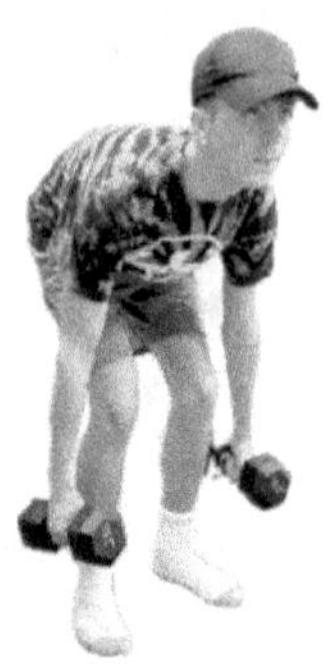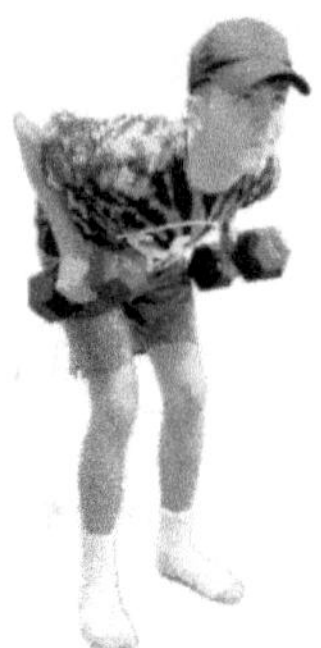

Hang power cleans - 10-20 reps every minute for 5 minutes:

1. First, stand tall with your dumbbells, holding them at your sides—hinge at the hips to lower them to your knees.
2. Then, stand back up with a slight jump, using the momentum to pull the dumbbells onto your shoulders. Stand up straight, then lower under control to your sides and repeat. Keep this fast and explosive; you're doing it wrong if your heart rate doesn't hit the roof.

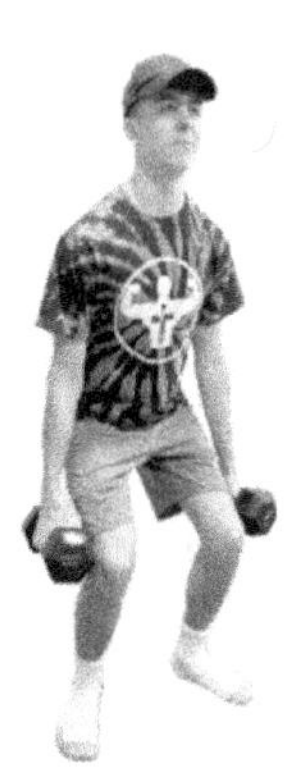 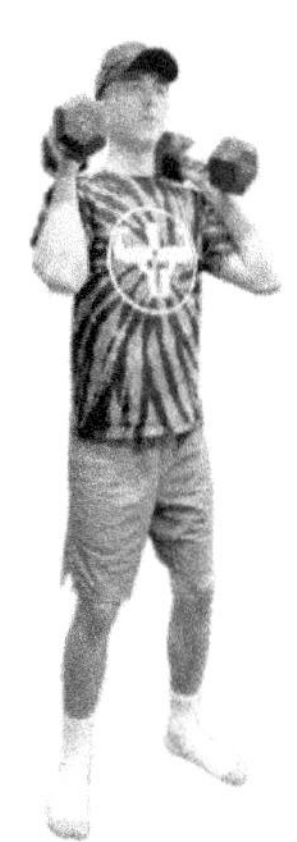

10

#3 The High Intensity Training Workout

Welcome to High Intensity Training 101. This workout is the only one of three requiring a gym membership or access to a multi-station home gym or universal gym. Unlike free weights, where moving the weight requires balance and movements in multiple planes, universal or weight machines provide movement over a fixed range of motion.

This workout was created from Doug McGuff's research and can be found in his fantastic book, "Body by Science." The workout takes anywhere from 12-15 minutes PER WEEK. Yes, you read that right. So now there is no longer an excuse for "I have no time to hit the gym." I have done this workout myself and trained my 73-year-old mother using these methods. It's hard to believe the gains in strength you can obtain with such little time in the gym, but if performed as Doug McGuff outlines in his book, you will also be a believer.

The four things you need for this workout are the five machines, a stopwatch (or smartphone with a timer), a progress chart (see appendix), a pen, and 110% effort for 12-15 minutes per week. The key to this

34

workout is extremely slow reps up and down for 90-150 seconds each set. McGuff calls "time under tension" (TUT) or the time your muscles are exerted with NO rest. The goal is to exhaust your muscles with each set. Remember that you only do 1 set Per exercise, so maximizing your effort is essential.

For example, the first rep may take as long as 10-15 seconds to complete, on the last rep you barely, if not at all, are moving the weights, but exhausting your muscles until you can't hold the weight anymore. You want to fail on each set. Slow repetitions, never locking out your arms or legs, never letting the stack of weights touch back down to the pre-start position, and not stopping the weight from moving (slowly). Keep your muscles working the entire set.

How much weight should you be using on each exercise? It may take 1-3 workouts to fine-tune it, but here are the two rules to help you figure that out.

- Rule # 1: If you cannot perform the set (repetitions till failure) for a minimum of 90 seconds or one minute and a half, you must reduce the weight until you can reach 90 seconds. Record the weight and times in your chart to know how to set up for the next workout.
- Rule #2: If you can perform the set (repetitions till failure) for more than 150 seconds or 2 1 / 2 minutes, you will increase the weight on the next workout.
- Rule # 3: Each rep is to be done slow in both directions, making sure to not pause in transition or rest the weights. The created the constant Time Under Tension to maximize your muscle exertion.

It's paramount to keep diligent notes on your weights and times right after each set or have your partner do it for you. The other key McDuff talks about is jumping from one set/exercise to the next within 10-15 seconds of completing the prior set. You activate your cardiovascular system by performing the exercises consecutively with little time between sets. Surprisingly, with this fast-paced workout, you may feel out of breath and sweat more than you would think. If you complete each exercise to failure as outlined above, with very little time in between, you will feel a great complete body pump, like you've been in the gym for an hour. It truly is a great workout. For more information on the science behind the workout, I recommend purchasing McDuff's Body by Science book and his BBS Question and Answer guide. Both are precious resources. You can also search Body by Science on YouTube for more videos on the workout.

The Big 5 Workout:

Seated Row

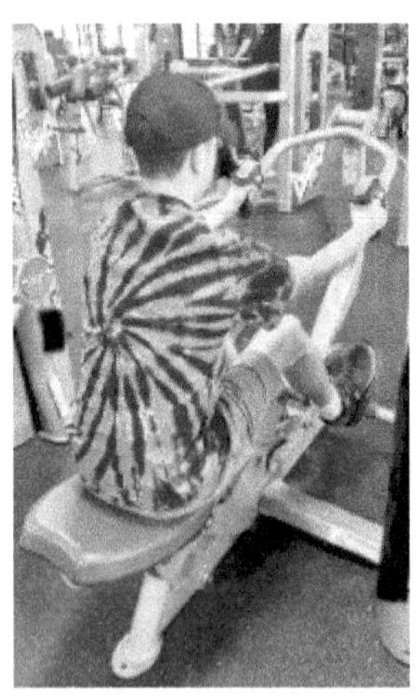
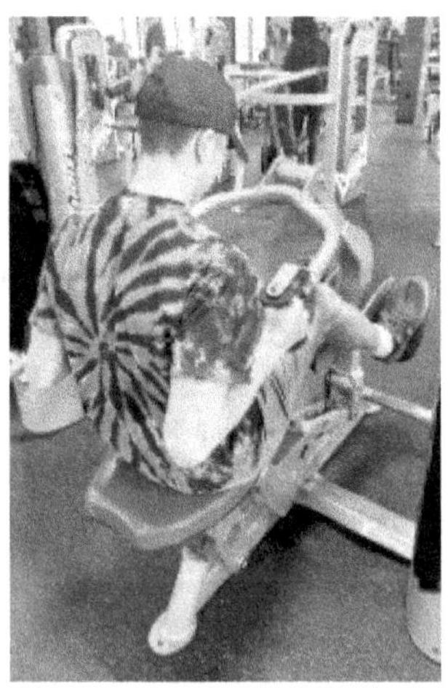

Chest Press

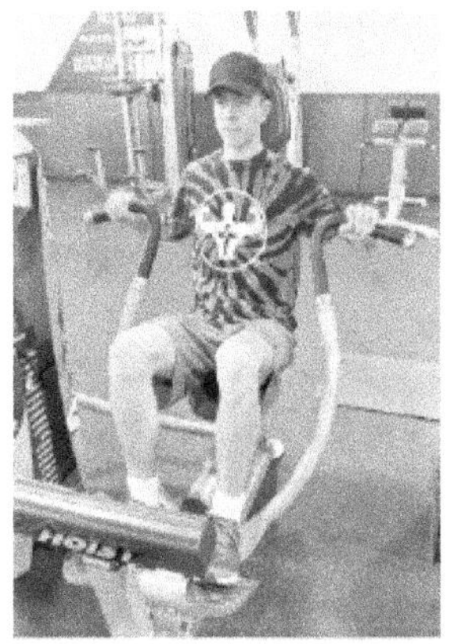 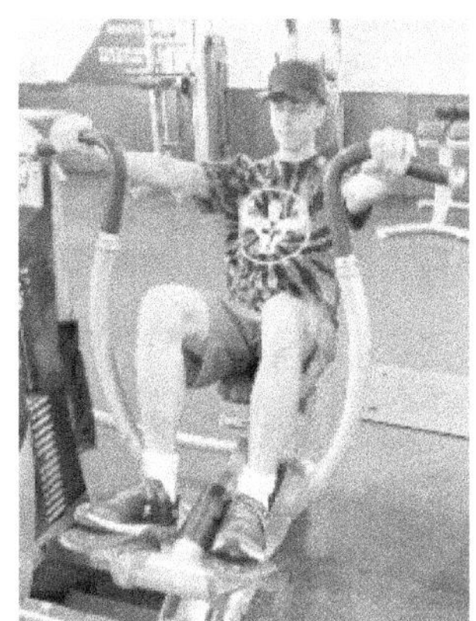

Lat Pull down

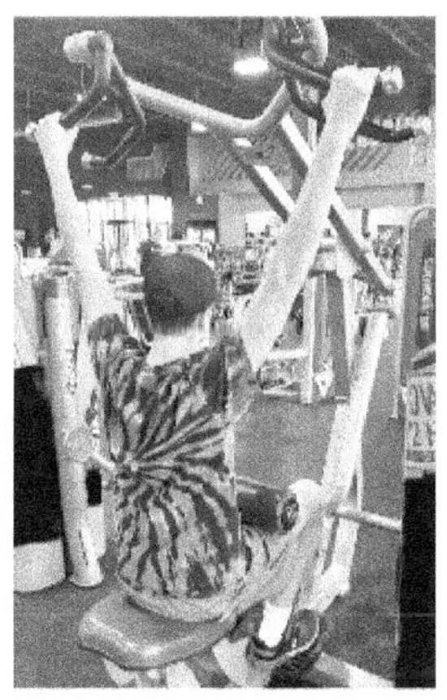 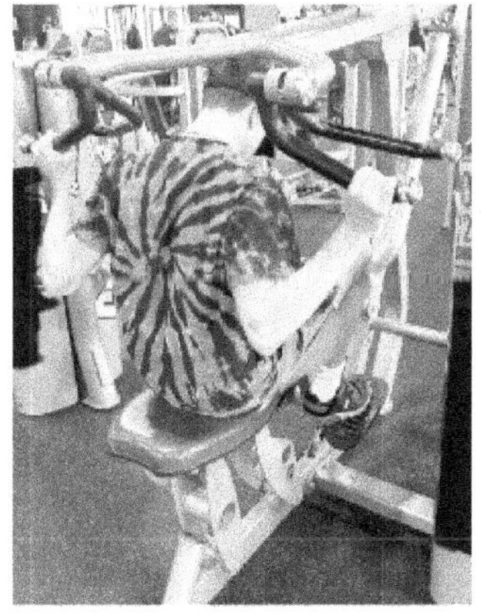

Shoulder Press

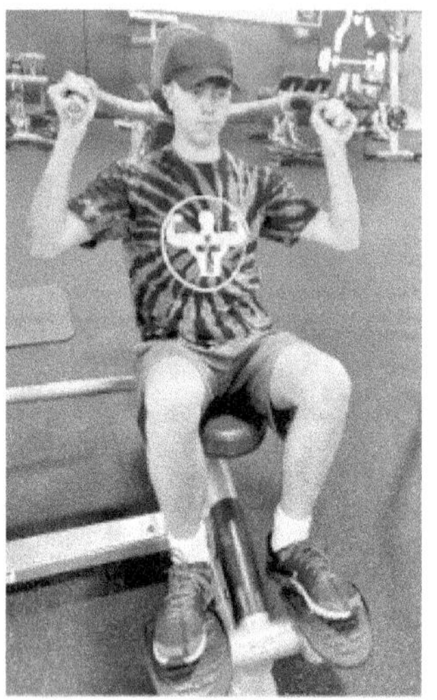 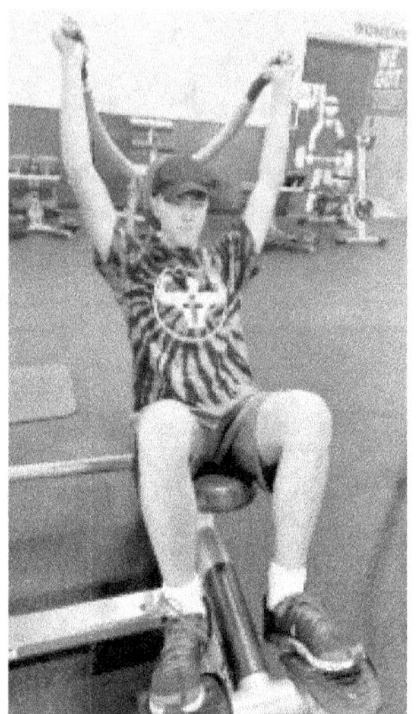

Leg Press

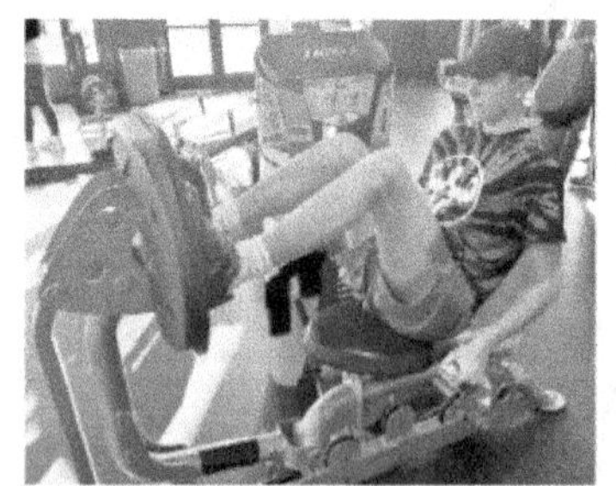 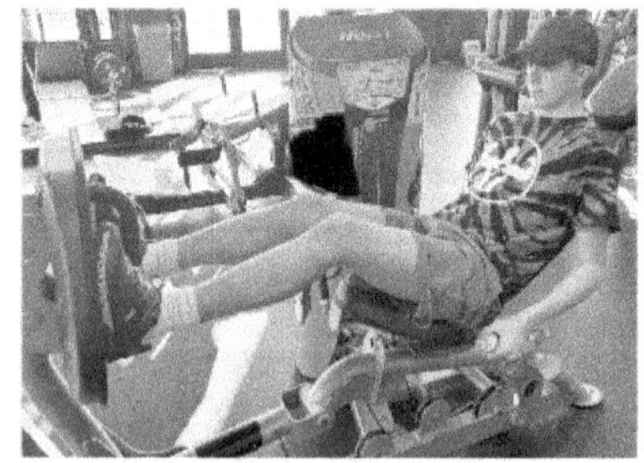

- See Appendix for the BBS chart you can print and track your progress.

11

Diet is important

Although starting an exercise regime is essential for health and longevity, I cannot stress enough how important diet is to your overall health goals. How much you eat is just as important as what you eat. I used to work for a Japanese company. One time when colleagues from Japan visited, I took them to lunch at a local sushi restaurant. When the waitress came to take our order, I ordered dumplings, edamame, a seaweed salad, and three rolls. They each ordered a Bento box, which is a single portion tray with usually four small servings of food. When I finished my lunch, they were still slowly enjoying their Bento box; I asked the waitress for the menu because I still had room in my belly. I ordered another specialty roll and asked my two colleagues if they wanted anything else. They looked at me with a wry smile and said matter-of-factually, "We only eat until we feel satisfied; you Americans eat until you are full." What a distinction and what an important lesson. Eat until you are satisfied, which is much easier if you steer clear of "all-you-can-eat restaurants.

There are so many schools of thought on what diet is proper. Atkins, paleo, vegan, the South Beach diet, intermittent fasting, etc... for now,

I'll give you the advice my mother told me for years. Eat in moderation. The word satiated comes from the Latin satiare, meaning "fill, full, satisfy," which is precisely how a satiated person feels — full and satisfied from a good meal. Unfortunately, in this country, we eat till we're ready to vomit. There are thousands of books written on healthy eating. Choose a diet that works for you, eat less than you need, and drink plenty of water. That's all I'm going to say about diet in this book.

12

Conclusion

After reading this short book, you will hopefully first and foremost realize YOU CAN DO THIS! You can fit a fitness regime into your busy lifestyle. You should now better understand your personal barriers, how to overcome them, and a few efficient workouts to get you moving within your busy schedule. These strategies include walking, body weight exercises, Micro workouts, and High-intensity training. You can start with one of these methods and add more complex and challenging training as you achieve your goals and milestones. Pick the ones that work for you, but the key is to start small and build on your new habits each day. The only way to succeed with these strategies is to keep going until this new habit becomes part of your lifestyle. It's easy for the slow pace of your visible progress (new body) frustrate you and make it easy to fall back into your bad habits. Keep working at it every week and over the long run you _will_ see the results.

Please keep track of your workouts (your data) because you won't know where you started or how you're doing without it. American Statistician and management theorist Edwards Deming said best: "In God we trust;

all others must bring data." If you found this book helpful, please leave a favorable review and share it with friends and family.

All my best, Maxwell "Max" Power…

Other Recommended Readings

1. **Body by Science**: A Research Based Program for Strength Training, Body building, and Complete Fitness in 12 Minutes a week. by Doug McGuff M.D.
2. **The Body by Science Question and Answer Book** by Doug McGuff M.D.
3. **The China Study**: The Most Comprehensive Study of Nutrition Ever Conducted and the Startling Implications for Diet, Weight Loss, and Long-Term Health. by T. Collin Campbell
4. **Atomic Habits**: An Easy & Proven Way to Build Good Habits & Break Bad Ones. by James Clear
5. **The Untethered Soul**: The Journey Beyond Yourself. by Michael A. Singer
6. **The Blue Zones Secrets for Living Longer**: Lessons From the Healthiest Places on Earth. by Dan Buettner
7. **The Four Agreements**: A Practical Guide to Personal Freedom (A Toltec Wisdom Book) by Don Miguel Ruiz

Resources

- *Why do people make excuses? 6 Mental Barriers to Fitness.* (n.d.). Gymaholic. https://www.gymaholic.co/articles/why-do-peopl e-make-excuses-6-mental-barriers-to-fitness
- *7 reasons why you should prioritize exercise during your everyday life | X Shadyside.* (n.d.). https://www.xshadyside.com/post/7-reasons- why-you-should-prioritize-exercise-during-your-everyday-life
- *Simple Body-Weight exercises to build your strength.* (n.d.). WebMD. https://www.webmd.com/fitness-exercise/ss/slideshow-bodywei ght-exercises
- Tracey, A. (2023, February 27). Could Ten-Minute 'Micro workouts' be the key to building the best physique of your life? *Men's Health.* https://www.menshealth.com/uk/building-muscle/a42939977/m icro-workouts/
- *Dr. Doug McGuff | Ultimate Exercise | Body by Science | Emergency Physician | Fitness Expert.* (2020, July 7). Doctor Doug McGuff. https://www.drmcguff.com/
- Zenhabits. (2022, April 18). *Overcoming Our Biggest Obstacle to Creating Habits - zen habits.* Zen Habits. https://zenhabits.net/ours elves/
- Solan, M. (2023, October 30). *How much sleep do you actually need?* Harvard Health. https://www.health.harvard.edu/blog/how-much -sleep-do-you-actually-need-202310302986#:~:text=Sleep%20qua lity%20counts%20as%20much%20as%20hours%20logged.&text=F

or%20most%20healthy%20adults%2C%20guidelines,least%20seve
n%20hours%20of%20slumber.

- Department of Health & Human Services. (n.d.). *Physical activity - how to get active when you are busy.* Better Health Channel. https://w ww.betterhealth.vic.gov.au/health/healthyliving/Physical-activity-how-to-get-active-when-you-are-busy
- Williams, P. T., & Thompson, P. D. (2013). Walking versus running for hypertension, cholesterol, and diabetes mellitus risk reduction. *Arteriosclerosis, Thrombosis, and Vascular Biology, 33*(5), 1085–1091. https://doi.org/10.1161/atvbaha.112.300878
- Tony, T. (2020, December 28). *7 ways to celebrate success | Tony Robbins.* tonyrobbins.com. https://www.tonyrobbins.com/mind-meaning/how-do-you-celebrate-your-success/
- *Fifteen ways to find more time in your day | Piedmont Healthcare.* (n.d.). https://www.piedmont.org/living-real-change/15-ways-to-find-more-time-in-your-day
- Eby, K. (n.d.). Free goal setting templates and goal tracking templates. *Smartsheet.* https://www.smartsheet.com/goal-trac king-setting-templates
- *5 Facts about Goal setting.* (2024, January). NEMOURS Teen Health. Retrieved February 20, 2024, from https://kidshealth.org/en/teens /goals-tips.html